THE ART OF MEDITATION:

How to Relieve Stress and Anxiety, Meditation for Beginners

Brian P. Davis

Table of content

Introduction for meditation

A mind-body technique used in complementary and alternative medicine is meditation (CAM). There are many different kinds of meditation, and most of them have their roots in lengthy religious and spiritual traditions. A person who is practicing meditation often employs certain practices, such as a certain stance, concentrated concentration, and an open mind to distractions. Meditation may be used for a variety of purposes, including to quiet down and relax physically, balance the mind and emotions, deal with sickness, and promote general wellbeing. This Backgrounder gives a broad overview of meditation and recommends some further reading.

Major Points

There are many health-related reasons why people meditate, but it is unclear what physiological changes take place during meditation if they have an impact on health, and if so, how.
Research is being conducted to learn more about the benefits of meditation, how it operates, and the illnesses and disorders for which it may be most beneficial.
• Be sure to let your medical professionals know if you practice any supplementary or alternative medicine. Give them a detailed account of your health management practices. This will help to coordinate and secure care.

Overview

A variety of practices are referred to as meditation, including mantra meditation, relaxation response meditation, mindfulness meditation, and Zen Buddhist meditation. The majority of meditation practices have their roots in Eastern spiritual or religious traditions. For thousands of years, many different civilizations throughout the globe have used these methods.

Today, many individuals practice meditation for health and well-being reasons outside of its traditional religious or cultural contexts.

Chapter 1

Meaning of Meditation

Relaxation, concentration, and awareness are all required for the mental activity of meditation. What exercise is to the body, meditation is to the mind. Individually, in a motionless sitting posture, and with eyes closed, the exercise is often performed.

What does psychology mean when it refers to meditation?
According to the definition of meditation given in psychology, it is "a family of mental training activities intended to acquaint the practitioner with certain kinds of mental processes" (source).

One of three different techniques is used to meditate:

concentrating one's mental or physical energy on a single thing (focused attention meditation)

Without allowing the attention to get fixed on anything, in particular, observation is paying attention to whatever is most prominent in your experience at the time (open monitoring meditation)

Allowing consciousness to stay in the present moment, unperturbed, and not involved in either focused or observing

Additional features of meditation include:

Even if it is done in a group, meditation is a personal discipline (such as in a meditation retreat).

Eyes closed while meditation is common, but not always (Zazen and Trataka, for example, are open-eye styles of meditation)

Body stillness is often required for meditation. However, there are various techniques for practicing walking meditation and incorporating attention into other tasks.

The term "mediate" originally meant to reflect carefully on something. However, for lack of a better phrase, this is the term that was used to designate eastern contemplative practices when they were "imported" to Western society. Nowadays, meditation is more often understood as a practice of attention-focus than as a time for in-depth reflection. Here are a few further explanations of meditation.

In Christianity, contemplative prayer, such as meditation, which cultivates a feeling of unity with God, or the consideration of religious issues, are both forms of meditation.

One of the three main techniques in Buddhism for clearing the mind and achieving Nirvana is meditation. Along with concentration, meditation calls for mental peace and introspection (or "gazing inside"). Thus, meditation differs slightly from other spiritual or personal development activities like:

In guided visualization, self-hypnosis, or affirmations, the goal is to imprint a certain message on the mind.

Pure relaxation, when the primary objective is to relieve stress from the body

When there is a deliberate flow of thought and emotion toward a Deity, it is called prayer.

Contemplation is the active use of one's mental processes to increase comprehension of a topic or idea.

Trance dancing, where the primary objective is often to induce hallucinations or a state of altered awareness

Exercises that concentrate on creating a certain breathing pattern and purifying the body include pranayama and (most varieties of) qigong.

While all of these approaches are beneficial and beneficial, they are not the same as meditation (although some meditation techniques may make use of some of these elements).

Chapter 2

Preparing for Meditation and how to meditate

Consider the goals you have for your meditation: People engage in meditation for a variety of reasons, including to enhance their creativity, assist in visualizing a goal, silence internal chatter, or establish a spiritual connection. It's sufficient to meditate if your main objective is to spend a few minutes each day in your body without thinking about all you have to accomplish. Don't make your motivations for meditation too complicated. At its essence, meditation is just about unwinding and avoiding daily worries.

Look for a quiet location to practice meditation: It's crucial to rid your surroundings of any distractions, especially when you're just starting.

Turn off the TV and radio, shut the windows to block off street noise, and lock the door to avoid rowdy housemates. Finding a calm area in your house where you can concentrate on meditation may be challenging if you live with roommates or relatives. If your housemates are willing to remain silent while you practice meditation, ask them to. Promise to let them know as soon as you're done so they can go back to their regular routines.

A fragrant candle, a vase of flowers, or some incense might be lovely finishing touches to your meditation.

To aid with concentration, turn the lights down or off.

Use a cushion for meditation: Zafus are an additional name for meditation pillows. A zafu is a spherical cushion that enables you to meditate while sitting on the ground. It does not allow you to slouch back and lose concentration on your energies as a chair does since it lacks a back. Any ordinary pillow or couch cushion will suffice if you don't have a zafu to prevent soreness over extended periods of cross-legged sitting.

Feel free to use a chair if you discover that sitting without a chair back bothers your back. For as long as it seems comfortable, try to keep your back straight. Then, lean back until you feel you can do it again.

Put on relaxed clothing: Avoid wearing constrictive apparel that can tug on you, such as jeans or tight trousers, since you don't want anything to wake you up from your meditative thought. Your best approach is to dress in loose, breathable clothing similar to what you may wear to work out or in bed.

Pick a time that is convenient for you: As you get more used to meditation, you could utilize it to soothe yourself when you're experiencing stress or overload. However, if you're just starting, it could be challenging for you to focus at first if you're not in the correct frame of mind. When you first begin, meditate when you are already in a state of relaxation, possibly right away in the morning or just after you have had time to decompress from school or work.
Before beginning your meditation, eliminate any potential sources of distraction. If you're feeling peckish, get a quick snack, visit the toilet if necessary, and so on.

Keep a timer close by: You want to make sure you meditate for a sufficient amount of time, but you also don't want to lose focus by looking at the clock. For whatever length you want to meditate—whether it's 10 minutes or an hour—set a timer. You can discover a lot of websites and applications that will clock your sessions for you, or your phone may already have a timer built in.

Ways to meditate

Straighten your back when sitting on your cushion or chair: Maintaining an upright position makes it easier to pay attention to your breathing as you deliberately inhale and exhale. Try not to slump or lean back against the back of a chair if it has one. Maintain as much posture.
Put your legs in whichever position seems most comfortable to you. If you're using a cushion on the ground, you may stretch them out in front of you or cross them underneath you like a pretzel. The most crucial thing is to maintain a straight posture.

Concerning what to do with your hands, don't worry. If putting your hands on your knees while meditating makes you uncomfortable, don't worry about it. We often see individuals doing this in the media. Whatever enables you to focus only on your breathing while clearing your thoughts is OK. You may fold them in your lap or let them dangle at your sides.

Tilt your head so that you seem to be gazing down: When you meditate, it doesn't matter whether your eyes are open or closed, however many individuals find that closing their eyes makes it simpler to filter out visual disturbances. In any case, cocking your head so it seems to be gazing downward will help you breathe more easily and open up your chest.

Start a timer: Set your timer for as long as you'd like to meditate after you're settled down and prepared to begin. Do not feel under any obligation to have a transcendental state lasting an hour in the first week. Start with short periods of 3 to 5 minutes, then work your way up to 30 minutes or even more if you'd like.

As you breathe, keep your mouth shut: When meditating, you should breathe in and out via your nose. Even if your mouth is closed, make sure your jaw muscles are at ease. Simply relax; don't clench your jaws or grit your teeth.

Remember to breathe deeply: This is the main goal of meditation. Give yourself something uplifting to concentrate on your breath. Don't attempt to think about the things that could stress you out daily. You'll discover that by concentrating just on your breaths in and out, all other ideas from the outer world will naturally fade away without you having to think about how to block them out.

Choose the breathing technique that feels most comfortable to you and focus on it: Some individuals like to concentrate on the movement of the lungs, while others prefer to consider the passage of air via the nose.

Perhaps you will concentrate on the sound of your breathing. Just go into a mental space where your attention is confined to one feature of your breath. Don't analyze your breath; just be aware of it.

Instead of being able to articulate it, the objective is to be present with each breath. Don't stress about remembering your feelings or being able to describe the event in the future. Simply take each breath in as it comes. Experience the subsequent breath after it has passed. Try to avoid thinking about your breathing; instead, simply enjoy it with your senses. If your focus leaves your breath, bring it back. Even after practicing meditation for a long time, you may still discover that your mind wanders. Later, you'll begin to consider employment, bills, or the errands you need to run. Never panic or attempt to ignore the outer world when you see it encroaching. Instead, slowly bring your attention back to the physical experience of breathing while allowing other thoughts to drift away once again.

It could be simpler for you to keep your attention on inhalations than on exhalations. If you discover it to be true, remember this. Focus in particular on how your breath feels as it exits your body.

If you're having difficulties focussing, try counting your breaths.

Be kind to yourself: Recognize that at first, it will be difficult for you to maintain attention. Don't criticize yourself; this inner dialogue is common among novices. Some even contend that this constant focus on the present is the "practice" of meditation. Furthermore, don't anticipate your life-changing as a result of your meditation practice. It takes time for mindfulness to take effect. Continue to practice meditation every day, extending your sessions by at least a few minutes.

Chapter 3

Types of Meditation Techniques

The Crucial Manual For Meditation

Exercises for a guided meditation that you may use anywhere, anytime.

An instructor guides you through the practice of guided meditation, either in person or via an app or course. Beginners should choose this kind of meditation since the teacher's experienced direction may help them get the most out of a novel experience.

Finding an instructor you enjoy and click with is key in this case while learning how to practice. Additionally, you may limit your search to a particular outcome and test out guided meditations that are geared toward acceptance, stress reduction, or sleep.

Mantra-based meditation

When practicing mantra meditation, you concentrate on a mantra, which might be a word, phrase, or syllable. This strategy is helpful because it offers your brain something else to concentrate on days when the ideas and emotions seem overpowering. Additionally, it is said to raise the vibrations connected to the mantra, assisting you in reaching a deeper and more upbeat level of consciousness.

How to exercise:
Pick a mantra that speaks to you. It might be a simple chant or a self-affirmation such as "I am worthy" (such as "om"). For a few minutes, repeat the phrase again and over. Don't worry about being sidetracked every time. Just return your attention to the slogan.

Prayer or contemplation

Spiritual meditation is the deliberate practice of having faith in and establishing a connection with something bigger, more expansive, and more profound than the human self.
By practicing this meditation, you are putting your faith in a higher power and the idea that everything occurs for a purpose.

How to exercise:

Repeat statements that encourage surrender and trust, such as "I am awake and aware," "I let everything just be as it is in this moment," or "I live in my Creator and my Creator lives in me," while sitting in quiet with your attention on your breathing.

Mindfulness meditation

We learn to shift from thinking to feeling via present moment (or mindfulness) meditation. This meditation enables you to become aware of your current surroundings or experience, importantly without passing judgment, as opposed to lingering on the past or dreading the future. It exhorts us to let our ideas be rather than to get emotionally invested in them.

How to practice: You can practice mindfulness meditation practically anyplace. Bring your attention to the physical breath and body sensations, such as the rising and falling of the chest and belly or the sensation of the breath as it enters and exits the mouth or nose. You might also concentrate on any nearby noises or odors. When you are comfortable, bring your awareness to your thoughts and feelings, allowing them to enter and then go. Think of your thoughts as ever-changing clouds drifting over a bright blue sky.

Using the vipassana method

This kind of meditation, sometimes known as "Insight Meditation," is sitting in quiet, concentrating on the breath, and taking note of any changes in the body or mind. The goal is to examine every facet of your life to get "insight" into the actual essence of reality, which vipassana theory holds is suffering. Vipassana retreats lasting several days are a well-liked method of deepening this practice.

How to practice: Take a quiet seat and focus on your breathing as it flows through your body. Allow all feelings, sensations, ideas, and noises to come without attaching yourself to them. Label any interruptions—for instance, "a bird chirping"—and then shift your attention back to your breathing.

Metta practice

This kind of meditation, often referred to as a "loving-kindness" meditation, involves bringing your consciousness to the people in your life—near and distant, known and unknown, loved and disliked—and sending them good vibes and thoughts. It's a fantastic method for taming anger and boosting optimism, understanding, and compassion.

How to practice: Sit comfortably and bring your consciousness to the center of your heart, with your eyes closed. Imagine that when you inhale, you are breathing in warmth, compassion, and unwavering love for yourself. As you exhale, visualize that you are sending that same warmth, compassion, and unwavering love outward to the people around you. Start with close friends or family members, then aim it toward neutral acquaintances, people you don't really like right now, and finally strangers.

The chakra technique

The seven chakras, or energy centers, of the body, are kept open, aligned, and fluid with the use of this meditation. It is predicated on the notion that by meditating on the chakras, we may restore balance to the self and heal any bad physical or mental conditions that may have resulted from blocked or imbalanced chakras.

How to exercise:
Learn about the chakras and the attributes that each one represents. Give the chakras that you believe require balancing some time to rest in your consciousness. Focus on where each chakra is located on your body and see the chakra's associated color's energy flowing through that spot. Here are some additional specifics on meditations created for each chakra's topics.

meditation in yoga
Yoga comes in a variety of forms, just as there are several varieties of meditation. Some, like Kundalini, emphasize the use of meditation practices to bolster and calm the nervous system. By concentrating on the breath and the present,

you may infuse any yoga style or class with a contemplative awareness.

How to practice: Focus your attention on your present-moment physical sensations and breath while doing any yoga pose. Every time you see your attention straying to other ideas, gently bring it back. One of the finest routes for meditation is corpse posture (savasana), which is done after every yoga session.

Candle-lit contemplation

Trataka, also known as candle gazing, is a kind of meditation in which you maintain an open gaze while concentrating on a single point or object, often the flame of a lighted candle. Crystals and other objects might also be utilized. This exercise may improve attention while assisting in bringing energy to the third-eye chakra.

How to practice: Take a comfortable seat and fix your eyes on a single thing, such as a candle, tree, or crystal. Try your hardest not to blink while maintaining relaxed eyes. Keep your eyes open until you start to feel uncomfortable, and then shut them. Keep the thing in your mind's eye, then open your eyes and begin the process once again.

meditation with visualization
During a visualization meditation, you focus only on seeing something or someone in your mind. Although it might seem difficult, concentrating on the breath or body is the same. By keeping them concentrated and giving them vitality, frequent visualization may assist you in achieving your goals in life.

How to practice: While comfortably seated and with your eyes closed, think about someone or something you either desire or have unfavorable sentiments towards and would want to let go of. Every time your thoughts stray, come back to this point and maintain your attention. Observe any potential physical feelings as well (such as body heat in response to anger). Do not get involved; instead, just keep watching.

Meditation when you only observe

Similar to vipassana, you bring your whole, unbiased awareness to the self throughout this meditation and take note of your thoughts, emotions, habits, and actions. You will start to understand yourself better via this concentration, and from that understanding, you will be able to make whatever changes you may need or desire to see in your life.

You may practice this meditation anytime, anyplace, by just turning your attention within. Observe your thoughts as though they were happening outside of you, being fully aware of your actions and ideas while staying objective and nonjudgmental. Keep a record of your experience.

The greatest effects will come from practicing meditation frequently, regardless of the method you use. Try a new approach every day for ten days, and then gauge your reaction. Also, keep in mind that you cannot meditate incorrectly, so relax if your mind is racing. That's perfectly typical. To allow oneself a little rest, meditation focuses on shifting focus and attention rather than trying to make the mind remain still.

Chapter 4

Daily life Meditation

Daily meditation the practice of staying present and mindful for a limited period can have numerous benefits for our mental and physical health. Yet, many of us don't meditate every day because we're too busy or we simply don't feel like it. Sound familiar?

The thing about meditation though is that we experience even greater benefits when we repeat the practice frequently and consistently. Finding some time each day to meditate even a short daily meditation is better than no meditation at all. Here's information and actionable tips to help you make meditation a part of your routine.

Science has proven that the benefits of meditation are too good to ignore. And while we don't need to meditate daily to experience its positive effect on our health and happiness, studies have shown that we can unlock even more benefits when we meditate for consecutive days. Completing just one 15-minute session of meditation using the Headspace app resulted in 22% reduction in mind wandering. And four weeks of using Headspace daily resulted in 14% increase in focus.

When we meditate, we can enhance our focus and decision-making and lessen our feelings of fear and stress. The result: by fundamentally shifting the way we relate to our thoughts and feelings, we can dial down the intensity of emotions that tend to take hold of us, and ultimately experience a greater sense of calm, clarity, and focus in our lives.

The particular benefits of daily generalized meditation are well-documented and widespread, ranging from reduction in anxiousness and lower blood pressure to increased immunity and better sleep. In a study that did not use the Headspace app, researchers from John Hopkins University found general mindfulness meditation programs helped ease psychological symptoms of depression, anxiety, and pain related to stress.

According to another study using a generalized form of meditation, people who meditate have lower levels of cortisol, a hormone associated with physical and emotional stress. Generalized meditation has also been proven to enhance sleep quality and, for people with chronic pain, increase pain tolerance.

What's more, individuals who meditate have also experienced benefits in their relationships, perhaps because meditation activates the portion of the brain connected with empathy. Three weeks of using the Headspace app was shown to improve compassion in research participants by 23%.

In summary, there are so many scientifically-backed ways meditation may assist your mind and body.

Try this brief daily meditation from Headspace

Start your free trial
How to start a regular meditation program

There's no way about it: developing a regular practice may help unleash even more advantages of meditating. Research suggests that frequency is even more significant than length — meaning, that meditating for 10 minutes a day, seven days a week is more helpful than 70 minutes one day a week.

Those individuals who are new to meditation — and even many who've been doing it for a long for that matter — find it tough to sustain a regular practice. That's why the "little and often" approach to meditation is so beneficial compared to solitary techniques we undertake once in a while and then leave behind. Committing to a short daily meditation helps your brain to learn at its speed how to be present in the here and now and how to extend that awareness to everyday tasks.

As with any habit, regular meditation gets simpler when it's part of your routine. Once it becomes a habit, we stop making excuses – we're too busy, we don't get anything out of it — and instead, we just meditate. So how can regular meditation become a habit that sticks?

Here's how to get started:

1. Decide on a time and location that works for you. One of the most effective methods to make your meditation practice into a habit is by striving to conduct it in the "same time, same place" every day. Many individuals like meditating first thing in the morning — before the day gets too hectic — because it sets them up for a focused day. But the greatest time to meditate is truly whenever you can best prioritize it. As for the perfect place? There isn't any. Simply, select a peaceful area to meditate where you feel comfortable and calm and distractions are minimized.

2. Decide on an amount of time to meditate. Particularly for beginners, beginning with short, manageable chunks of time — for example, 3, 5, or 10 minutes — is crucial so you can build up your practice and discover your sweet spot (which differs for everyone) (which varies for everyone). The most essential thing is to select an amount of time that is beneficial, but still seems doable and

keeps you motivated. That's the only way you'll keep turning up day after day. Research reveals that pairing a 30-second activity with a "habit anchor" might make new habits more likely to persist. The 30-second activity might be anything that can motivate you to start your new daily meditation program (For example: "I will count 15 inhales and exhale breath cycles for 30 seconds before I start meditating"). And the habit anchor is something you currently perform as part of an established daily routine that you can tie that new 30-second activity to (such as "I will begin counting my breaths as soon as I finish brushing my teeth").

3. Make yourself comfy. Choose a meditation position that feels pleasant for your body. This might be sitting in a chair or on a sofa with feet flat on the floor, kneeling, legs crossed on a hard cushion or yoga mat, laying down on your back, or even standing or walking. If you're seated, try to maintain your back straight, your hands resting on your lap or knees, your eyes looking quietly into the middle distance or at a point on the floor in

front of you. Posture might be helpful for attention, but, feeling comfortable is more vital. So, feel free to select whichever posture seems best for you (also, know that this position might vary depending on the day) (and, know that this position could change depending on the day). Comfortable clothing are good, and you may even wrap a blanket over yourself if you tend to feel chilly when sitting motionless if that seems more comfortable.

4. Use a guide, such as an app. A guide or a guided meditation program like the Headspace app may be a valuable, accessible tool for creating a regular meditation practice. Most meditation applications are geared for both beginning and seasoned meditators and give useful education, insights, and support on several themes.

Headspace includes various tools that might help you start a regular meditation practice and put you on the road towards a better, healthier life. The run streak feature logs the number of days you have meditated in a row. Seeing how regularly you've been working toward your goal might help keep you on track with meditating helping you follow through on your purpose and commitment to a daily meditation practice.

Everyday Headspace is another beneficial aspect, especially for individuals who want variation in their practice. Delivered to your phone and available on the Headspace app home screen, it's a daily meditation on a new theme each day. There are also super-short meditations you can conduct on those days when you can only get in a minute or two. And of course, Headspace provides hundreds of themed meditations with configurable lengths on anything from sleep and anxiety to mindful eating and self-esteem.

When you're ready, hit play on Headspace's 10-day beginner's course on mindfulness essentials accessible with your subscription or free trial. Jump into your new practice with the necessities.

Chapter 5

How Medication Relieve Stress and Anxiety

How can meditation ease stress?

It offers us the room to figure out which demands on our energy, attention, and emotions are legitimate and which are not. Just think—if we could discern between the two, our experience of stress and anxiety would be quite different. We feel pressure when we don't have this space in our thinking and our lives. We sense relief when meditation offers us the space and clarity we need to order our priorities. This is the demand side part of stress management.

Mindfulness meditation is also a wonderful foundation practice for stress avoidance so that when unpleasant conditions arise we don't allow them to go out of hand.

Stress prevention

We all endure stressful experiences in life, such as the death of a loved one, divorce, or relocating, all of which are considered high-stress occurrences. Any event of this kind—or even just hard conditions at work—demands a lot from us, therefore we would be prudent to understand some fundamental strategies to react to stressful situations that cannot be avoided. During those key periods in our life, meditation may assist bring solace. How? By providing us a greater understanding of how to interact with circumstances, a heightened awareness of our emotions, and more room to react. For example, when we mourn for someone, the more conscious we are of everything that is going on in our brains, the better we can handle our pain and grief. When we're not conscious, our emotions tend to tint our vision and judgment and inflate our impression of what the circumstance asks of us, so that it is believed to be beyond what we think we can supply. This is the insidious cycle of stress.

Managing anxiety with meditation

Understanding anxiety is the first step in controlling it. In comprehending its irregular character, we may get a better awareness of triggering events and how our anxiety acts — and that's where meditation comes in.

Anxiety is a cognitive condition associated with an inability to manage emotions. But research suggests that a continuous meditation practice reprograms neural connections in the brain and, consequently, increases our capacity to manage emotions.

Through meditation, we acquaint ourselves with anxiety-inducing ideas and stories. We learn to notice them, sit with them, and let them go. In doing so, we discover 2 key things: ideas do not define us, and thoughts are not real. Within this unique viewpoint, we're able to progressively shift our relationship with worry, discerning between what is an illogical episode and what's genuine.

Another advantage of this ability is acquiring body awareness, which enables us to draw our attention to any bodily feelings encountered in the present. This approach entails mentally scanning the body, inch by inch, making us more receptive to what's being experienced physiologically. In investigating these experiences, we sit with our senses in the same way we sit with our ideas. This go-to strategy may give a secure spot that can be frequently visited anytime fear begins to seep in.

Try 7 meditations for anxiety

Looking for more meditations to feel calmer and less worried? The Headspace app provides users various courses and solo meditations on reducing anxiety, including:

- Managing Anxiety course. Cultivate a different viewpoint on fear.

- Bring Yourself Back video. Use this practice to generate greater mental space from worrying about things that haven't occurred yet.

- Reframing Anxiety exercise. Find a place of calm by carefully releasing the tension, one muscle at a time.

- Worry counsel. What do we do when worry develops during meditation?

- Awake Worrying evening SOS. Ease your mind by practicing the loving-kindness approach toward yourself and your loved ones.

- Mental Chatter midnight SOS. Create the space for the mind to softly come to rest with this bedtime meditation.

- Deep breathing exercise. A restorative session with special concentration on the breath is perfect for returning you to a more centered, quiet mind.

Chapter 6

Benefits of Meditation

1. It lowers cortisol levels. Research shows that mindfulness meditation lowers levels of cortisol, the hormone that causes stress. Reducing cortisol

can decrease general stress, anxiety and depression.

2. You can better deal with stress. Meditation brings a sense of calm to the mind and body that can reduce stress, Washam says.

"When the mind relaxes and lets go, the body follows," she says. "We want our adrenaline and our nervous system to take a break at times, to unplug, to recycle, to rejuvenate."

3. It eases anxiety. "Meditation is literally the perfect, portable anti-anxiety treatment," says health coach Traci Shoblom. Taking just a few minutes to close your eyes and do breathing exercises can turn off the mechanisms in your brain that cause anxiety

4. It reduces depression symptoms. Depression is a series mental health condition often triggered by stress and anxiety. Research suggests meditation can change areas of the brain, including the "me center" and "fear center," that are linked to

depression. People who meditate also show increased gray matter in the brain's hippocampus, responsible for memory.

5. You'll get a mood boost. Meditation helps you deal with stress, anxiety and difficult situations, which makes you happier and feel better. "We're just able to deal with difficult things without letting it affect your mood," Washam says.

Serendipity

6. You can retrain your brain. The brain tends to develop as it's used. Meditation may retrain the brain to use the prefrontal cortex, known as the "me center," to regulate the amygdala, or "fear center," says researcher and author Bracha Goetz.

"This means that when faced with a stressor, when we are not meditating, we will have gotten in the habit of using our prefrontal cortex to direct our minds back to think more calmly and clearly focus, rather than letting our impulsive reactions direct us," Goetz says.

7. It's good for your heart. Research shows meditation can reduce the risk of cardiovascular disease, says Chirag Shah, physician and founder of online healthcare platform Push Health. Meditation positively impacts blood pressure, heart muscle effectiveness and general cardiovascular mortality.

8. It lowers blood pressure.High blood pressure affects about 30% of U.S. adults and is considered a worldwide epidemic that heightens the risk of stroke and heart attack. Meditation may improve blood pressure naturally, without medication, research shows.

9. It enhances serotonin levels. Serotonin is a chemical produced in nerve cells that works as a natural mood stabilizer. When you meditate, you'll increase serotonin levels, which Washam says acts like a natural anti-depressant.

10. You'll break bad habits. Whether it's smoking or shopping too much, meditation brings awareness to your actions in that moment and help you break the cycle of a bad habit, Washam says.

Most habits form unconsciously, she says, and, "Over time, (meditation) brings awareness to what we're doing, so we're not acting out unconsciously. Mindfulness interrupts the habit."

11. You'll strengthen relationships. Good communication, empathy and respect are the hallmarks of a strong relationship, and meditation helps improve all of those qualities. Creating a deeper connection with yourself makes relationships easier and more fulfilling.

12. It boosts concentration. When so many things are racing through our minds at any given time, it can be tough to concentrate on tasks at work or even hobbies like reading a book. Meditation centers your mind so you can focus on what you need to get done.

13. It helps build inner strength. We've all been stuck in traffic or in a long, boring meeting and couldn't wait to escape. Practicing meditation and mindfulness helps build inner strength and endurance to calmly get through these situations, Washam says.

"It creates an ability to be in the moment no matter how it is," she says. "We're just able to be with difficult things without unraveling or letting it affect you."

14. You'll learn to be present. Research shows meditation can decrease brain activity in the default mode network (DMN), the part of the brain that wonders, worries and overthinks, helping us stay in the present, says Adina Mahalli, relationship expert and mental health professional at Maple Holistics.

"Meditation promotes being in the present moment and focusing our thoughts," Mahalli says, explaining that meditation works the brain like a muscle. "The more you meditate the more easily you're able to snap out of DMN mode and into the present."

15. You'll become comfortable in stillness. These days, most of us are always on the go and rarely take the time to calm down. Meditation can make you feel comfortable with stillness, says Josee Perron, life coach and yoga and meditation teacher.

"We've become accustomed to needing to be on the go all the time," Perron says. "But, so much running around doesn't leave any time for stillness, which is the gateway to connecting with your deeper inner self."

16. It helps with brain fog. If you struggle with concentration, forget things easily and have a hard time focusing, you might have brain fog. It's often caused by stress, and a meditation practice can

calm your mind and let you focus on your breath so you feel more present.

"Meditation cuts through the fog because we're waking up in that moment in a way, literally," Washam says. "We're stopping the habitual distraction, which has effects in the brain long term."

17. You'll better handle anger. Getting angry is a natural feeling when dealing with difficult people or situations. If you act impulsively, you could make things worse, however. When you meditate, you train your brain to focus on the present, and this can help you learn to control and process your emotions in the moment.

"Maybe you're upset, but you slow down and just feel your emotions," Washam says. "Just that simple act of turning toward your breath creates a kind of relief in the mind."

18. You can work through grudges. Holding onto anger and reliving past wrongs in your mind takes a toll on the mind and body. To calm these feelings, Washam suggests using STOP, a mindfulness–based meditation technique, which stands for stopping in the moment, taking a breath, observing your internal feelings and proceeding with your day.

19. You'll live in the moment. Learning to focus and live in the moment is an important benefit of meditation, but it's easier said than done. Often, our thoughts turn to past events or things we need or want to do in the future, and we seem to forget about the here and now.

20. It helps you cope with pain. Meditation activates areas of the brain that are associated with processing pain, so mindful breathing can help people manage chronic pain, says Megan Junchaya, health coach and founder of Vibe N' Thrive. Research shows that even a short amount of meditation can boost pain tolerance and reduce

pain-related anxiety—and, it could possibly
alleviate the need for opioid pain medication.